Praise for
Being with Heart

"The art in this book is beautiful, mysterious, whimsical, complicated, simple, and captivating. Each illustration is, in itself, like a story, or a poem, or a love letter. The brief text feels like a heartfelt gift of love from the author to the reader. I turned the pages again and again with joy and gratitude. It is impossible to describe the feeling this book leaves you with."

—E. Bluestein, author of *Tea and Other Adam Na Tales*, winner of the G.S. Sharat Chandra Prize for Short Fiction

"Art and writing that is inspiring and heartfelt."

—Esteban Utreras PhD

"*Being with Heart* is a love offering from Pascale Dellefield to the world. The vibrant illustrations and pithy sayings on connecting to the heart are accessible across a wide range of ages and abilities, a reminder to us all to stay present with love and gratitude."

— Louise Julig, past director, San Diego Shambhala Meditation Center

"*Being with Heart* touched my heart. There is love in every word and in every painting."

—Georgine Brave, Esq

More Books from
The Sager Group

Students Write the Darnedest Things: Gaffes, Goofs, Blunders and Unintended
Wisdom from Actual College Papers
by Pamela Hill Nettleton, PhD

Big Noise from LaPorte: A Diary of the Disillusioned
by Holly Schroeder Link

Meeting Mozart: A Novel Drawn from the Secret Diaries of Lorenzo Da Ponte
by Howard Jay Smith

Lavender in Your Lemonade: A Funny and Touching COVID Diary
by Chris Erskine

Sarabeth and the Five Spirits: A Novel about Channeling, Consciousness,
Healing, and Murder
by Mike Sager

The Deadliest Man Alive:
Count Dante, The Mob and the War for American Martial Arts
by Benji Feldheim

Lifeboat No. 8: Surviving the Titanic
by Elizabeth Kaye

The Pope of Pot: And Other True Stories of Marijuana and Related High Jinks
by Mike Sager

See our entire library at TheSagerGroup.net

BEING WITH HEART

How to
Thrive in Life
with a Tender Heart

Written and Illustrated by
Pascale Dellefield

Published in the United States of America.

Cover and interior art by Pascale Dellefield
Cover and interior designed by Siori Kitajima, PatternBased.com

Cataloging-in-Publication data for this book is available from the Library of
Congress
ISBN-13:
eBook: 978-1-958861-11-0
Paperback: 978-1-958861-12-7

Published by The Sager Group LLC
(TheSagerGroup.net)

BEING WITH HEART

How to
Thrive in Life
with a Tender Heart

Written and Illustrated by
Pascale Dellefield

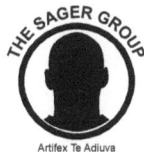

THE SAGER GROUP

Artifex Te Adiuva

Being with Heart is a journey of transformation. It is a reminder of the true resilience of our hearts. When we stay connected with our tender hearts throughout life's ups and downs, we uncover our deepest feelings, and the true strength within.

For Ken

List of Illustrations

Blissful Heartful Dancer

All Weathering Heart

Noble Heart

Dribble Up

Growing Up

Brave Heart

Swans in Love

Eye in the Sky

Anchor in Time

Never Lose Heart

Elephant Call

Bridge the Gap

Angel Full of Heart

Bright Side

Upright in Heart

Blindspot

Heartful Flower Phoenix

Foreword

I wrote *Being with Heart* because I wanted to have a part in healing the world emotionally, as a way to cultivate awareness that ultimately paves the way for heartfelt presence, healing and peace. It is my hope that *Being with Heart* will take readers on a journey of self-discovery by illustrating a myriad of ways to stay open and available to nurturing one's own heart at all times.

Guiding readers with colorful, child-like illustrations, *Being with Heart* is a gentle reminder to all of us that our heart is resilient and can burn to ashes countless times and then awaken to rise like a phoenix. In our world today when we get hurt we build walls in our attempt to protect our hearts. *Being with Heart* encourages us to be brave and kind. We are asked to keep our hearts tender and wide open and to trust that our wounded hearts can heal and recover.

In *Being with Heart*, I try to show readers how to stay present with their hearts. By doing so, they will find themselves more able to open their minds to all experiences in life, be they painful or joyous, and to do so lovingly. The book stresses the importance of staying open and reveals how essential it is to live in the world with a mindset of compassion.

Given the challenges of our times, both children and adults are finding it more and more difficult to stay present and mindful while opening their hearts. It is my hope that these whimsical, simple, and colorful drawings take readers on an emotional and psychological journey that helps them to grow and mature, and to be open to the delights and joys of seeing the world with all its magic.

It is my hope that *Being with Heart* is relevant to readers of all ages. Though it is a slim book, take your time with it. It is filled with colorful symbolic illustrations accompanied by brief descriptions as well as short poems that are easy to remember. The book offers profound life lessons and wisdom. Once the reader has completed the book from front to back, something magical may happen in the heart center, as the reader begins to understand what it is to experience *Being with Heart.*

—Pascale Dellefield

Keep in touch with your beating heart at all
times.

Whole or in pieces,
keep your heart close.
After all,
you only have
one heart

Uncover its deep feelings –
hearts love that!
It's how they feel loved.

Along the way,
as your heart beats,
pounds,
or gently pulsates,

and as life
pulls,
pushes,
and
cradles you,

wear your heart
with courage

and let your heart feel
all the pains and joys.

This is the same way
that nature works
with sunrise and sunsets.

Keep your heart
running like a clock.

Make sure you don't lose it,

avoid it,
hide from it,
misplace it,

or let it escape from you.

The surest way to keep your heart
and keep it healthy

is to stay with your heart
present

with Love

and Gratitude.

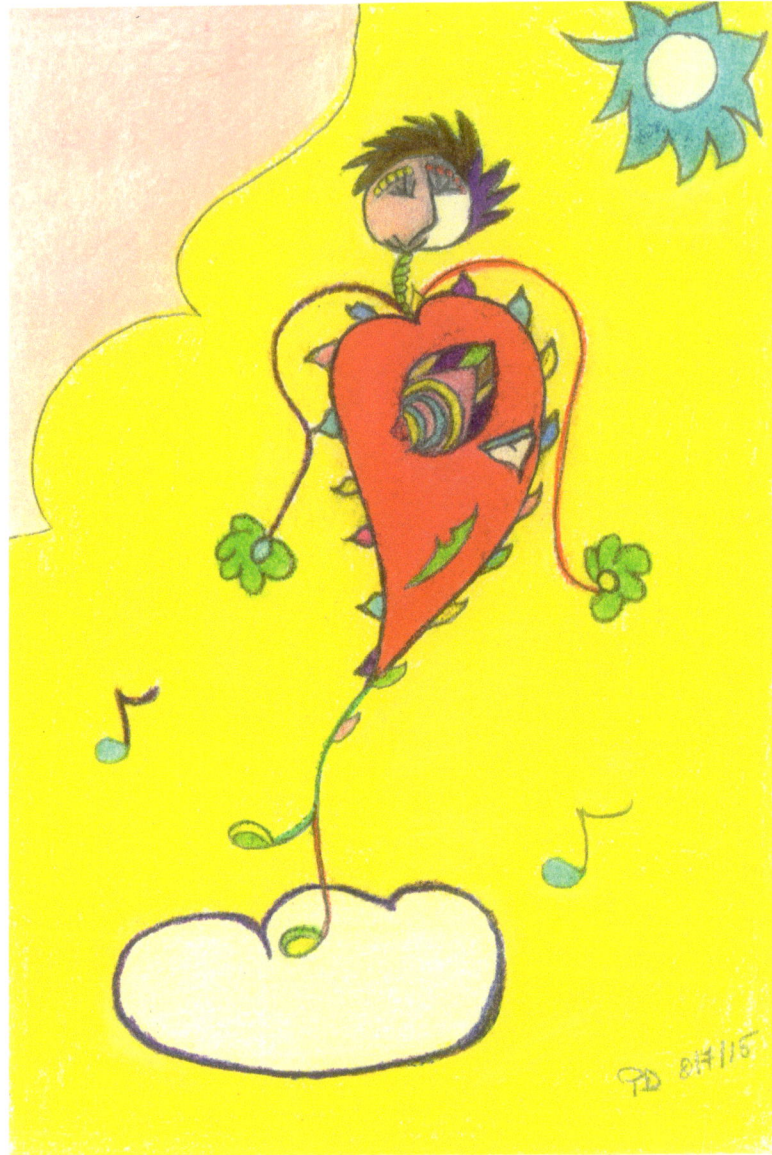

Blissful Heartful Dancer

Dance in the moonlight
Let your music stem from love
Find joy in your heart
And let it spread and glow

When you step in a puddle or a cloud, plant
yourself in your heart. Let the joyful music
that stems from your heartbeat spark joy in
two musical notes on your feet, two flowers
in your hands, two squints of bliss in your
eyes, and a splash of purple on the edges of
your hair.

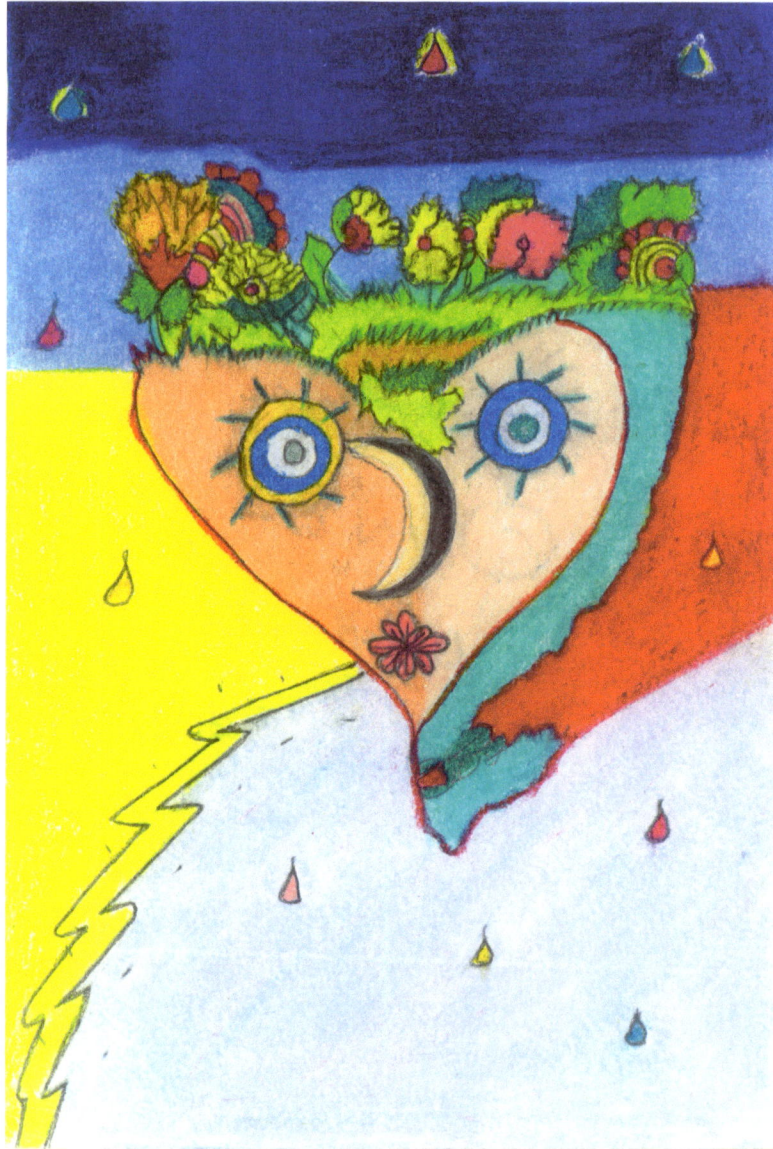

All Weathering Heart

All Weathering Heart
Weathers any conditions
My heart awakens

During trying times, let love breathe, grow, awaken you, and guide you, and you will see your heart has unconditional love that can weather all conditions.

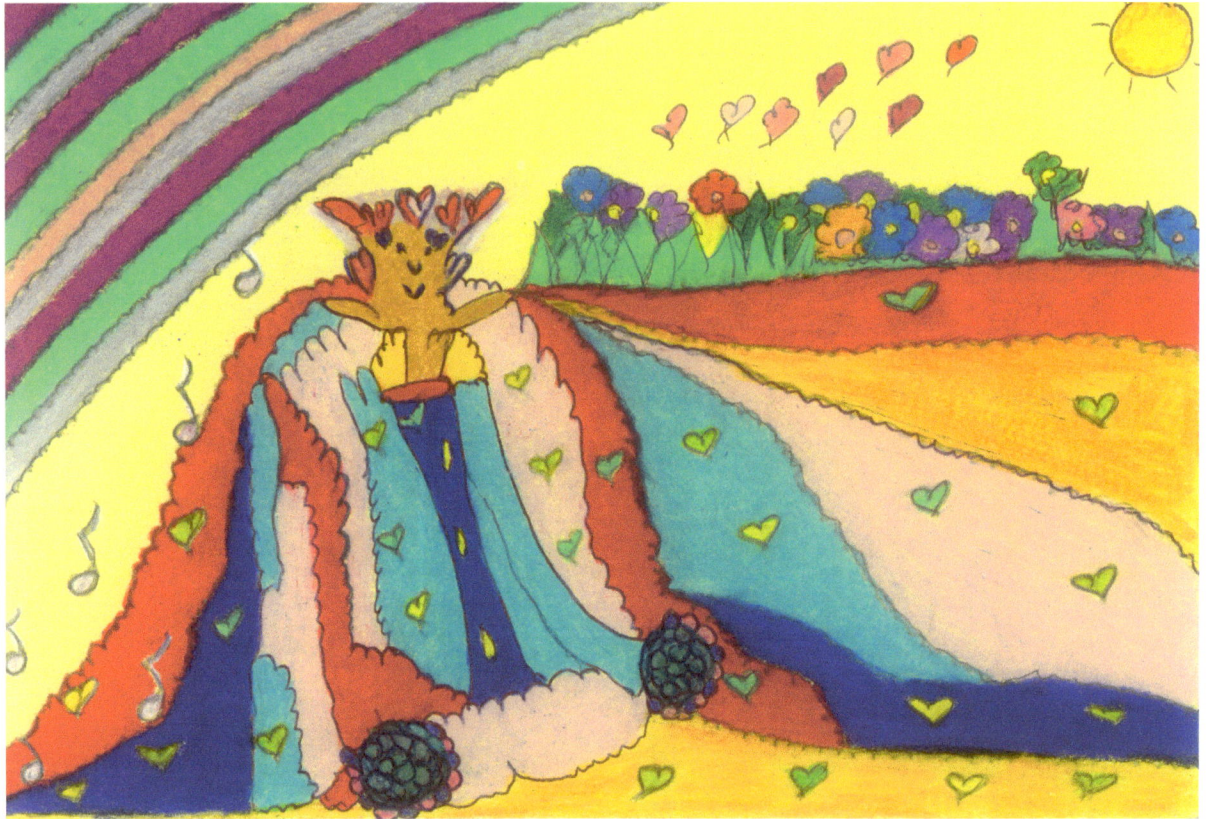

Noble Heart

Joy blossoms
In a realm of compassion

When you are blessed with a position of authority or power, let love rule, reign, spread, and shine. Celebrate it under a crown of service to others with ears full of Love and fists full of flowers.

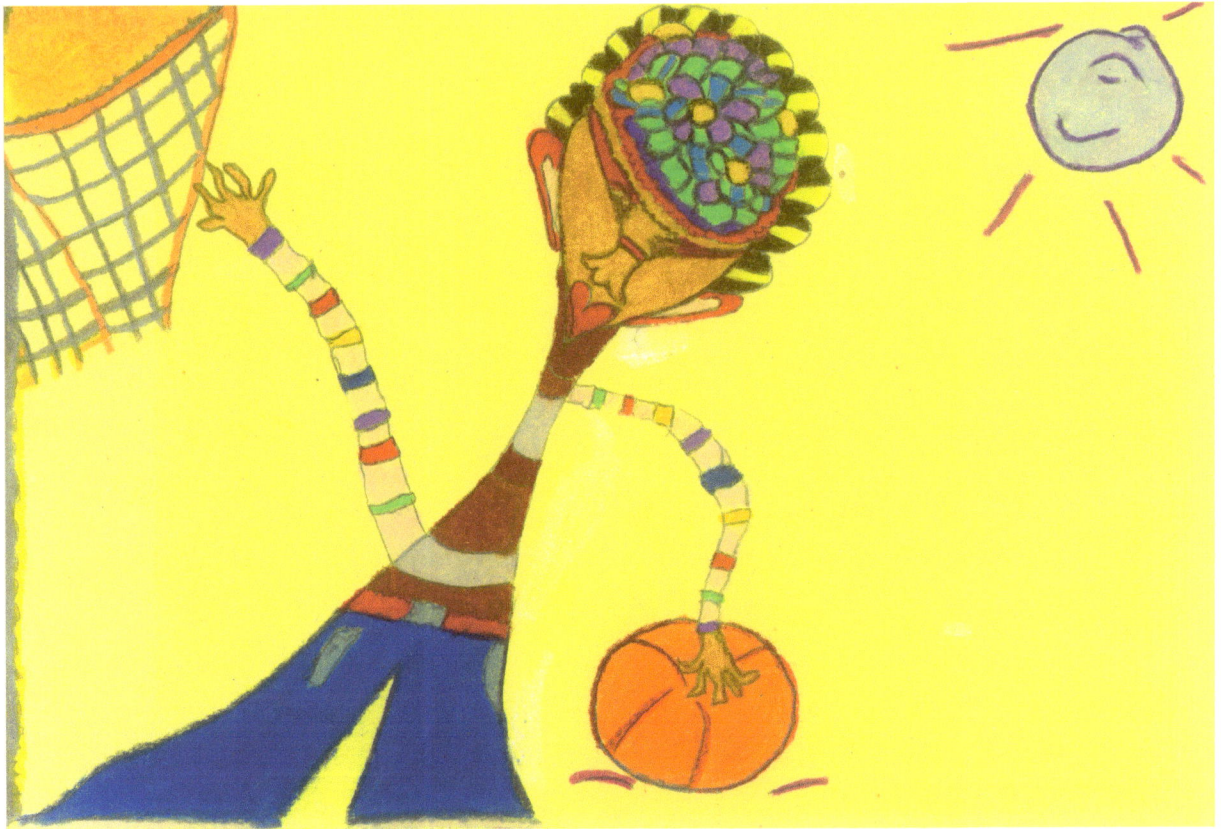

Dribble Up

Get out in the sun
It's time to have fun

Light up your brain, think like the bees, speak from the heart, practice your steps to dribbling, reach out and network, and you are nearly there, with your goal at your fingertips.

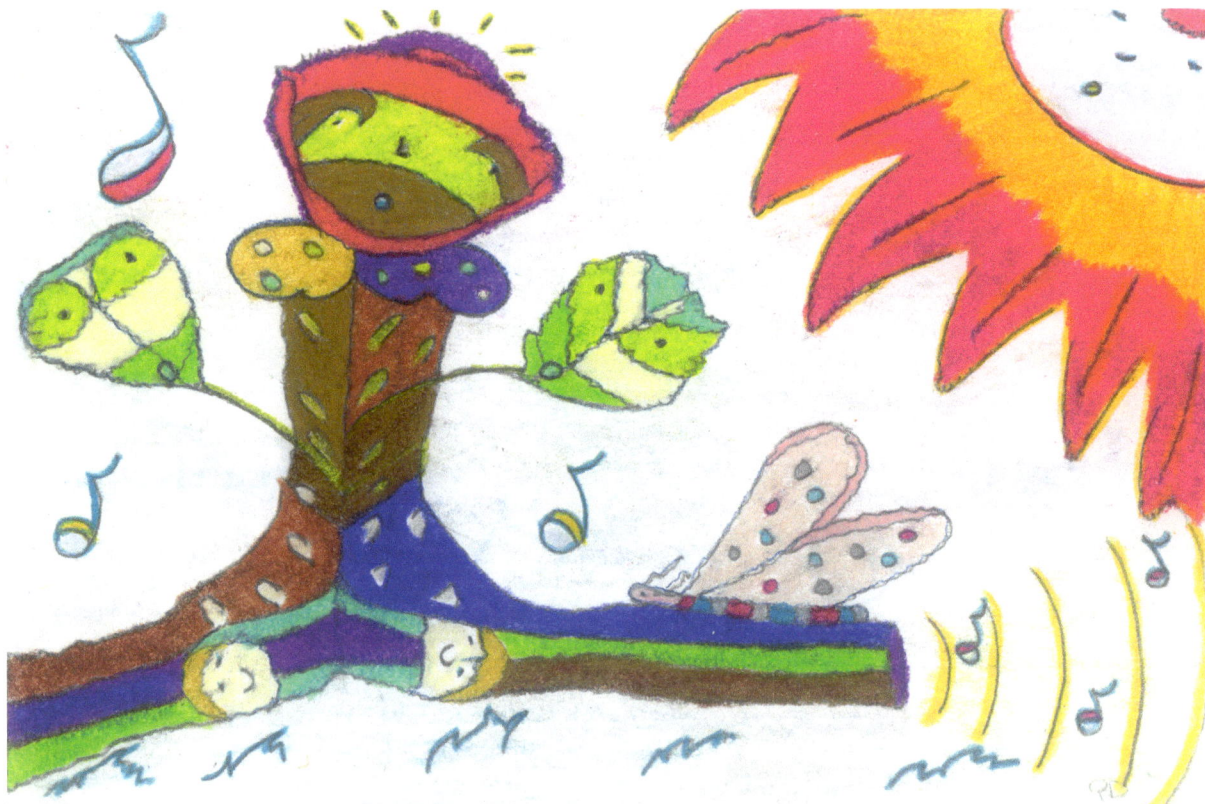

Growing Up

I tune my ears
towards the ground
And raise
my wingbeat vibration
Then face the music
with open arms
And once I tie up in a bow
my head over my shoulders
It's time to tip my hat
And bask in the sun

When you are up a stump, it's time to grow
up and let go, keep your ear to the ground,
spread your wings, branch out from your
trunk, tie up the bow, and continue in harness.
Then tip your hat to the sun.

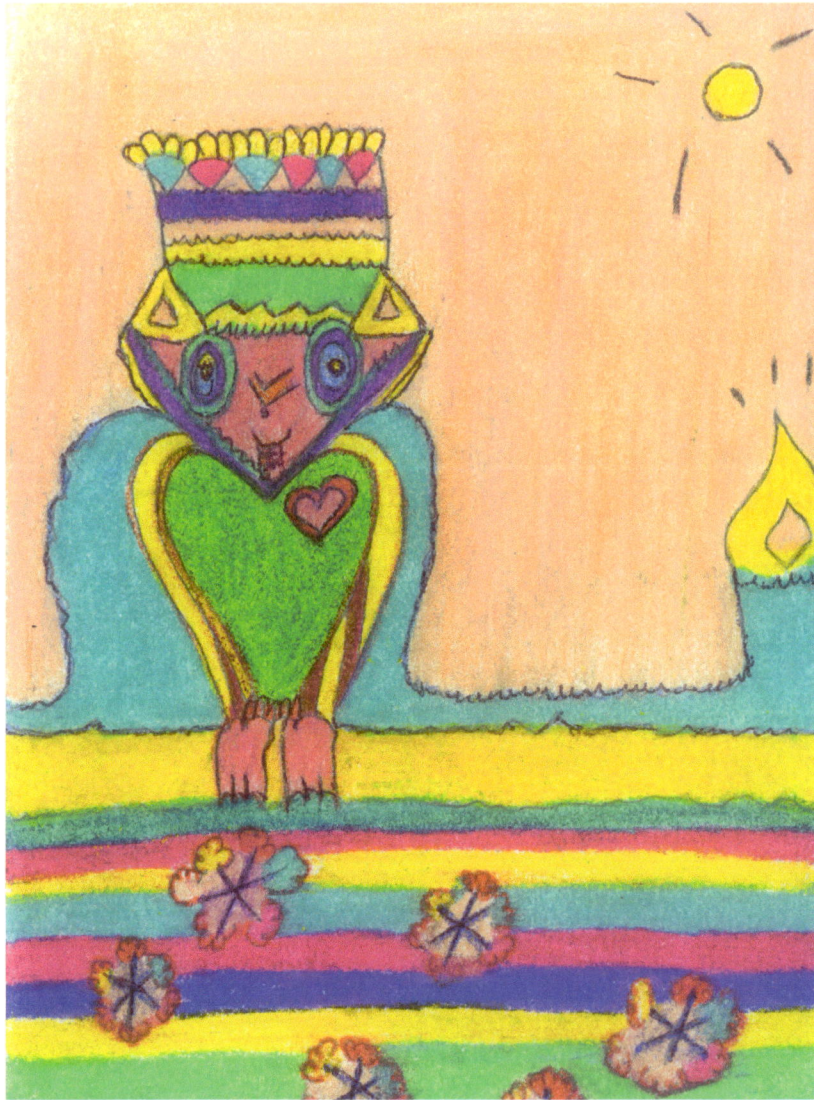

Brave Heart

Love burns
day and night
When my crown is lit
with birthday candles
to Celebrate
my brave heart
Another year

When your burden feels heavy and your heart
feels too small to carry it, remember the
crown on your head is a cake adorned with
birthday candles, lit from the love in your
heart that burns day and night.

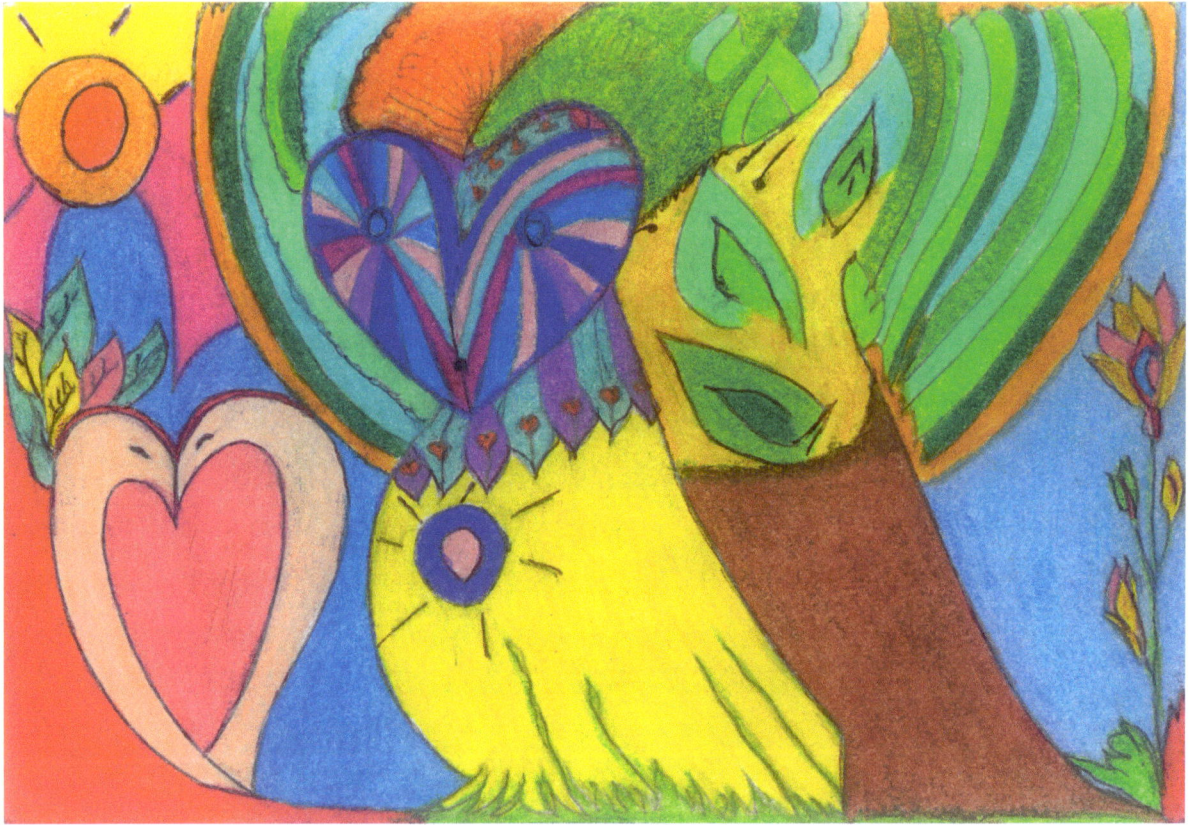

Swans in Love

Find your heart center
The place where
your heart is soft
And Trust
that the love
in your heart
is primordial

When love seems out of reach, lean into your
heart and trust that when you have light in
your heart, and your heart is lit, love will
appear in your life.

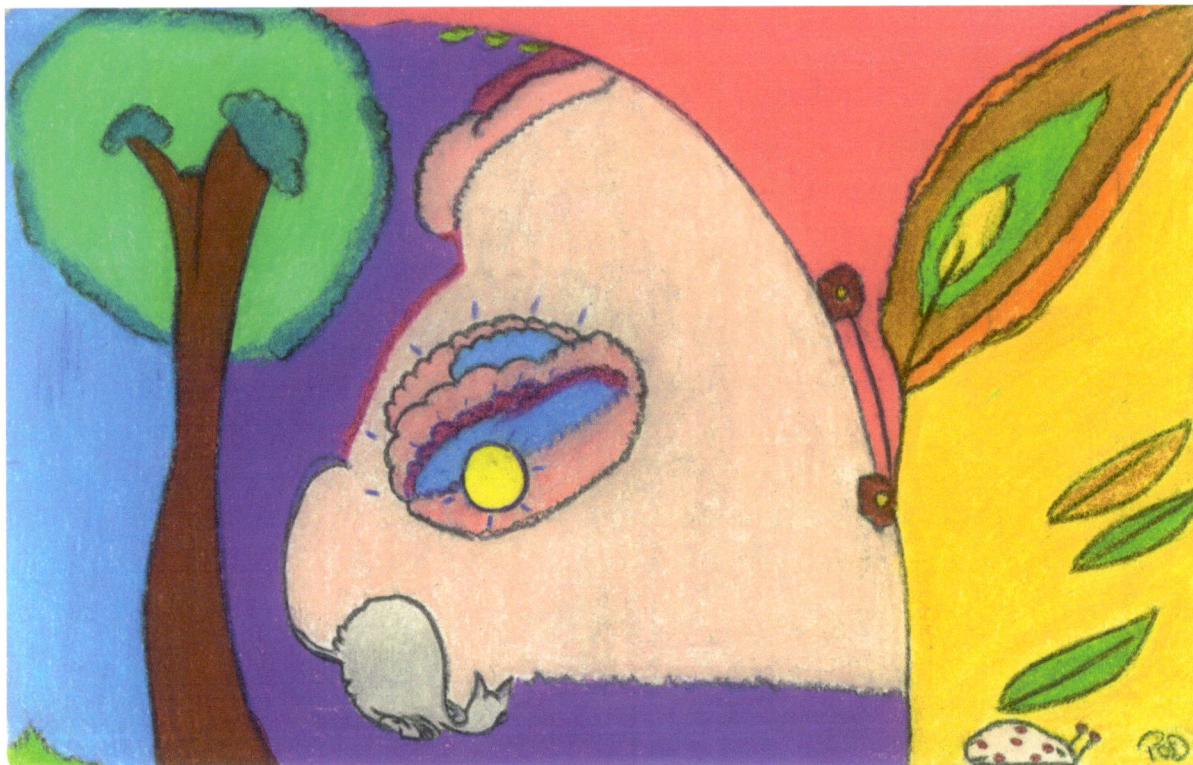

Eye in the Sky

Have faith in life
One day at a time

When you are skittish like a cat, or are worrying
about your next meal, like a ladybug —See
the eye in the sky, and trust that the universe
will provide.

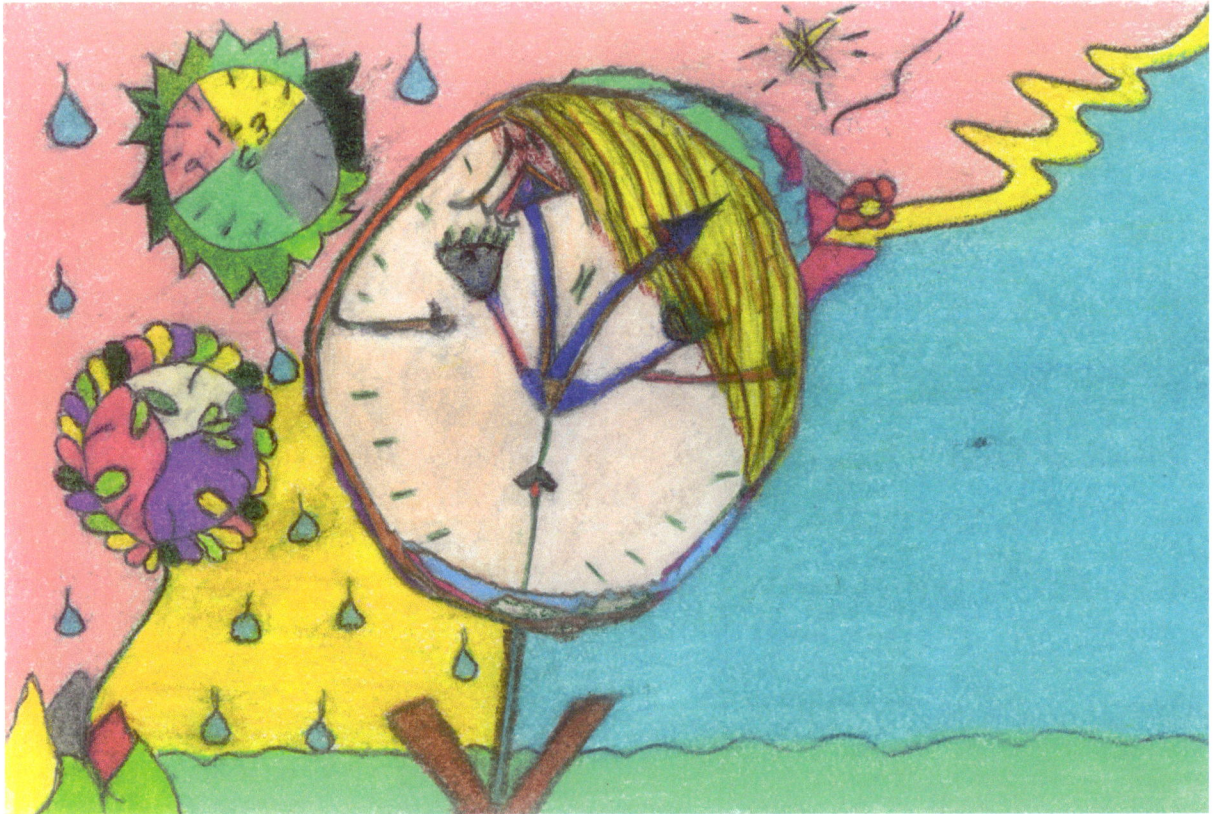

Anchor in Time

Meditate
Time is a present

When lightning strikes out of the blue, drop
an anchor in the present. It's time to wake
up.

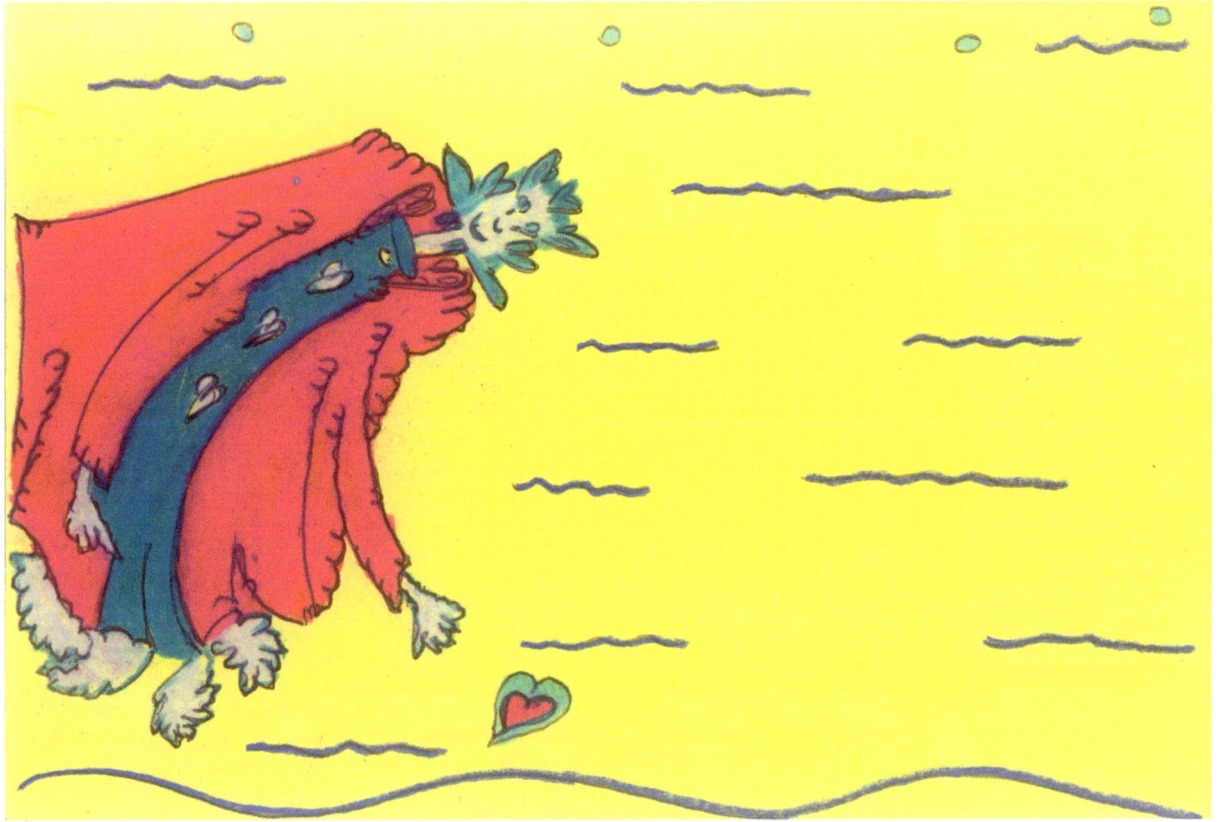

Never Lose Heart

Keep a head above
the level of the heart
Keep a level head
And never lose heart

When you find yourself with your heart to
lose, keep a level head, and your head above
the level of your heart.

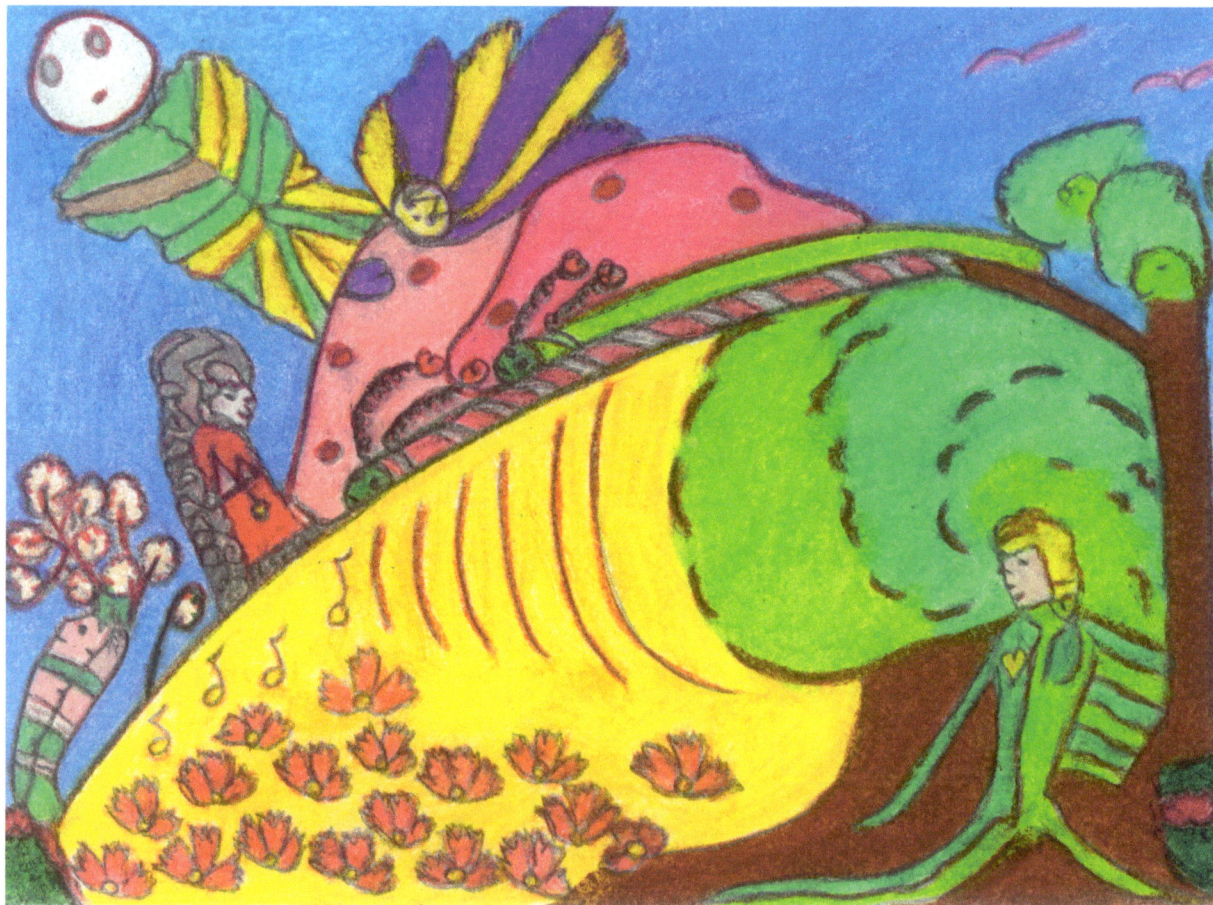

Elephant Call

When you hear the Elephant Call
It's time to spread love
into a wood wide web
And reach for the moon
Where we can achieve
world peace

When the world seems divided, headed in the
wrong direction, or losing its way, broadcast
an elephant's call from your heart, spin your
love into a wood wide web, and together
from one generation to the next, reach for
the moon.

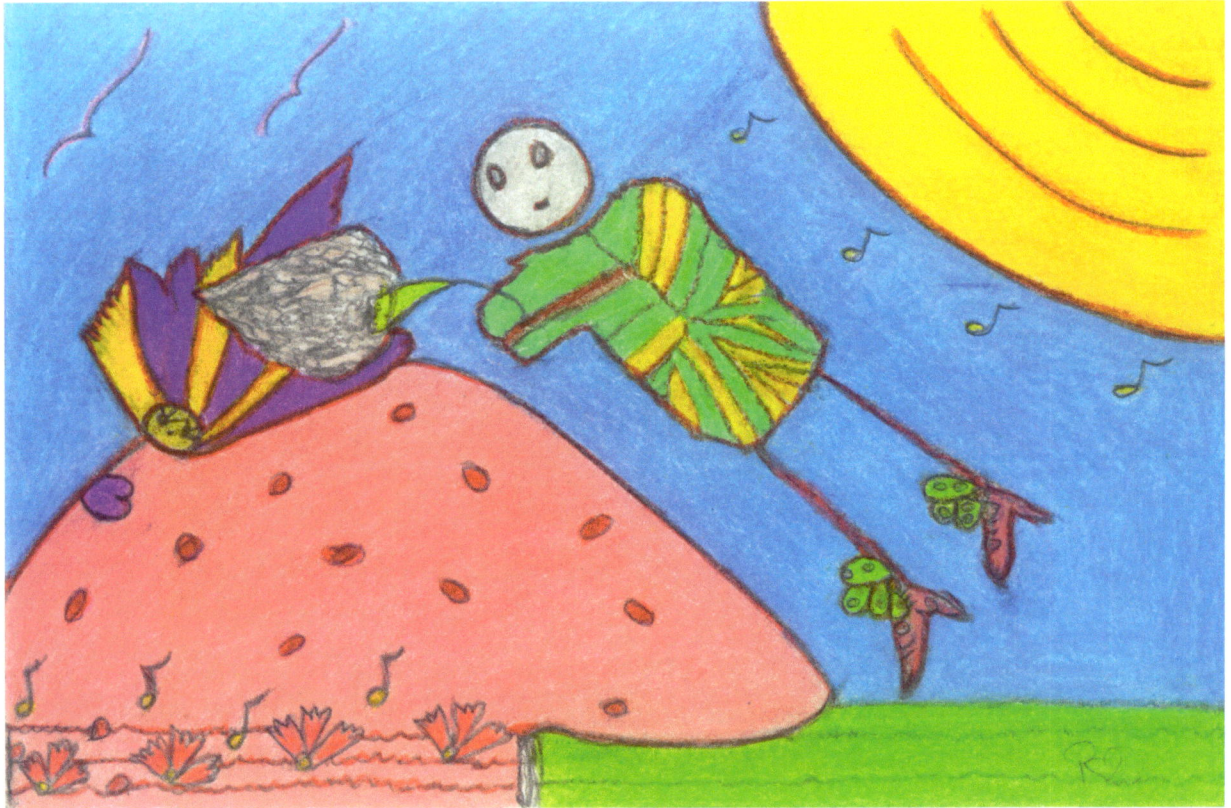

Bridge the Gap

Earth belongs to no one
and everyone
Bridge the gaps of differences

When you feel uprooted like the birds in the
skies, migrate, plant seeds in the earth that
will bloom like flowers in the sunlight and
bear the fruits of your love by the light of
the moon.

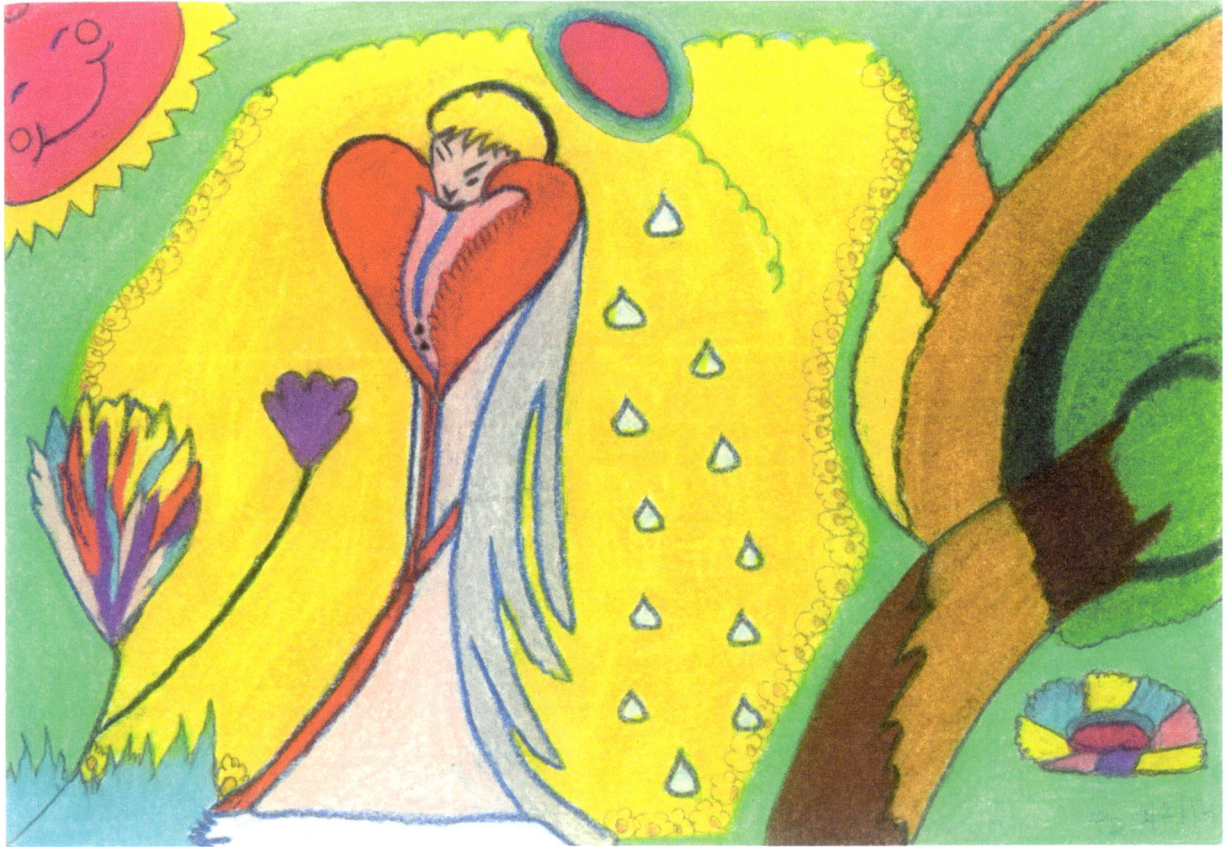

Angel Full of Heart

Get back on the path
Of the heart of compassion

When tempted to stray from your heart
conscience, let your head bow to your heart,
and love hold you in the light.

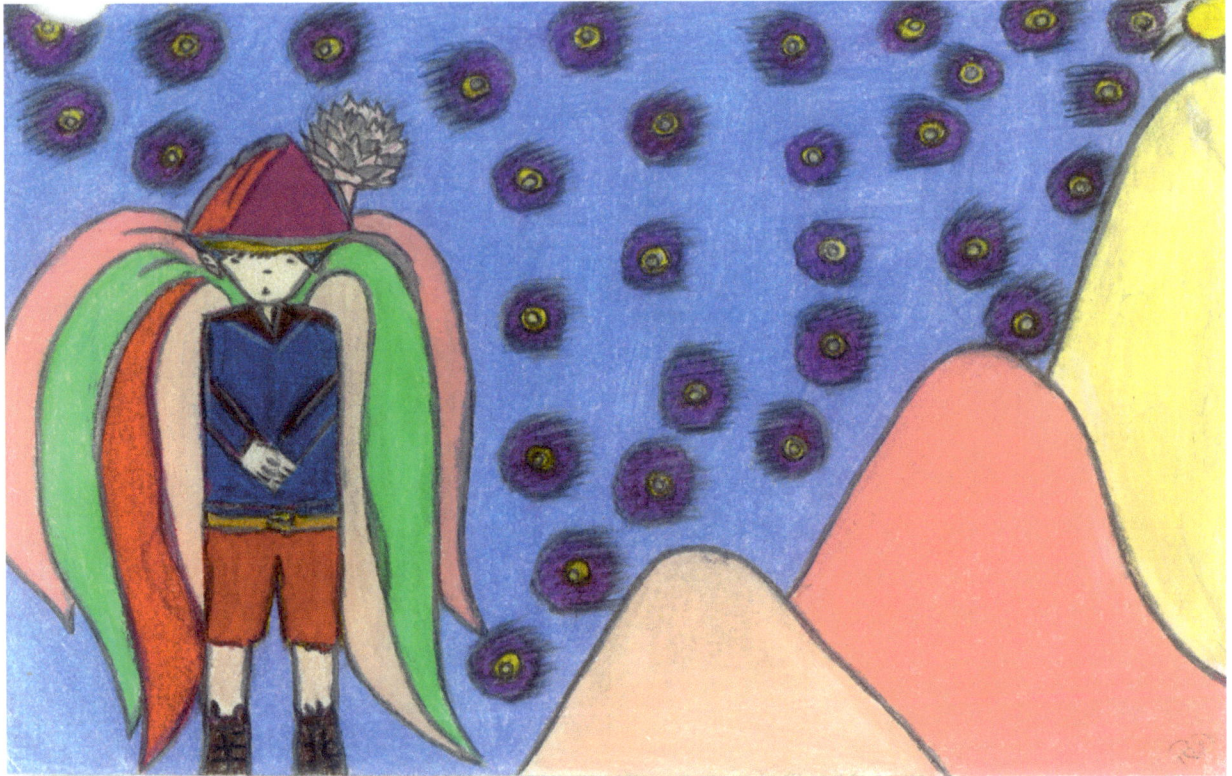

Bright Side

Existential fears
When life expires
And death arrives
Love with all your might
And fear not in your heart

In your darkest hour, silversword angel,
when it's snowing far below zero, and you
are feeling wing-weary, remember to look
up and notice the bright light in the dark,
behind the highest mountain peak.

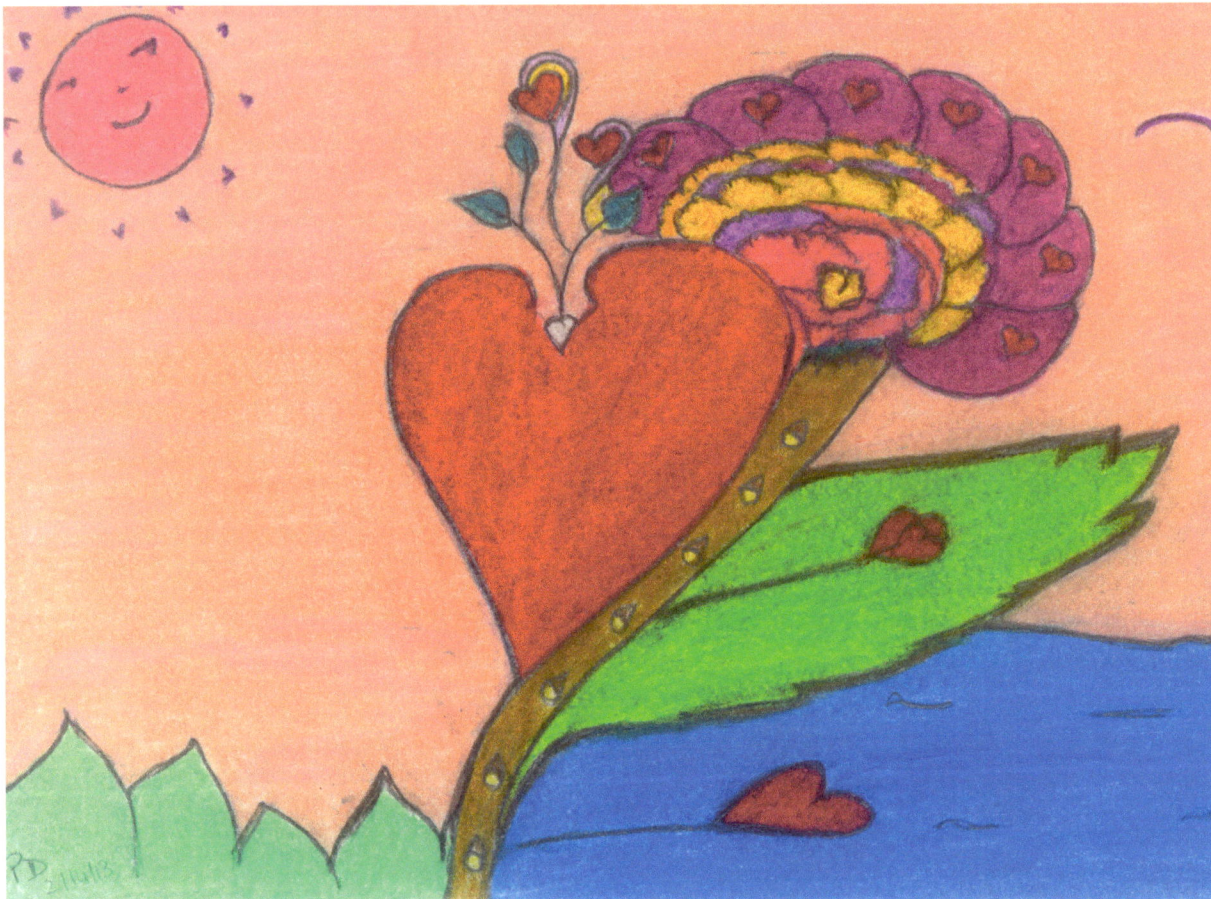

Upright in Heart

Rise above
the changing tides

Be upright in your heart and turn the tide.

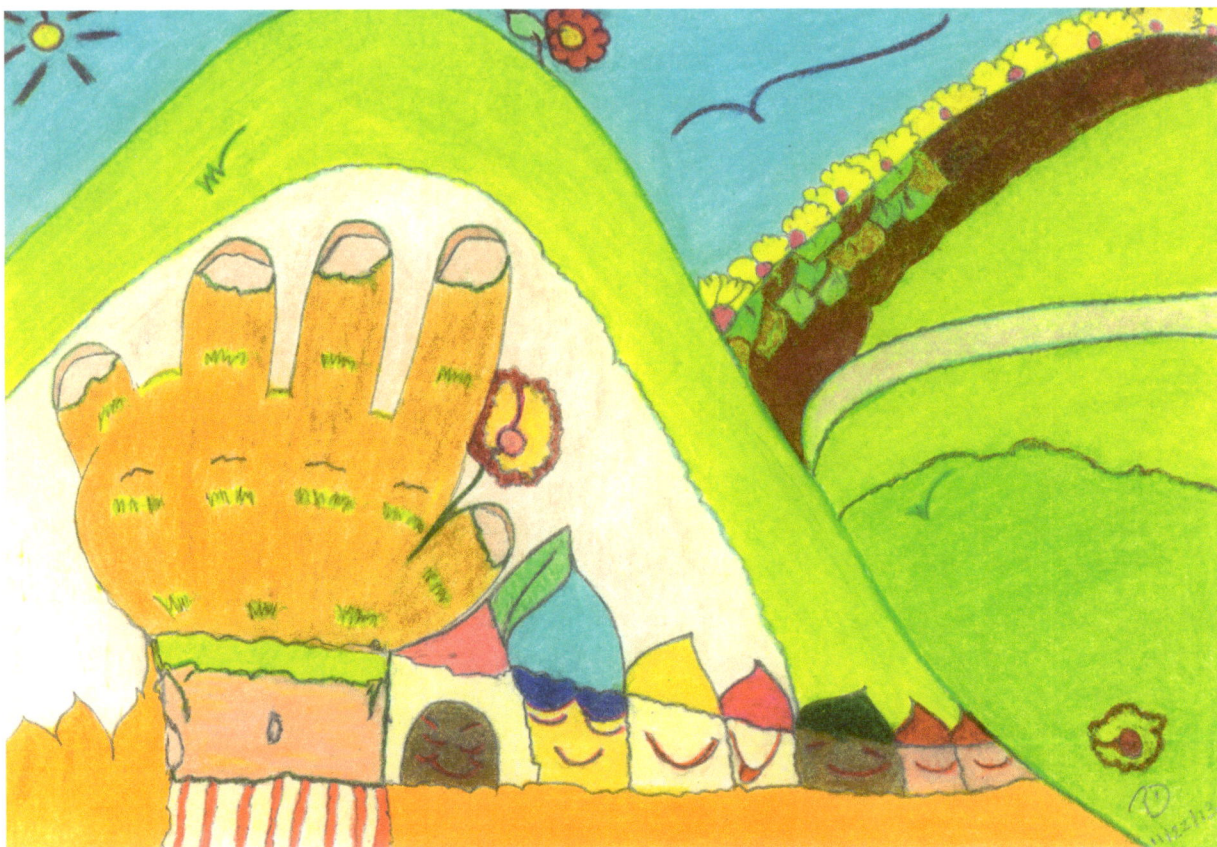

Blindspot

Trust what your heart knows

When your blind spot seems as large as a mountain and you are unable to see what's in front of you, take your hand off your blind spot, and remember to trust your heart to understand the picture perfectly.

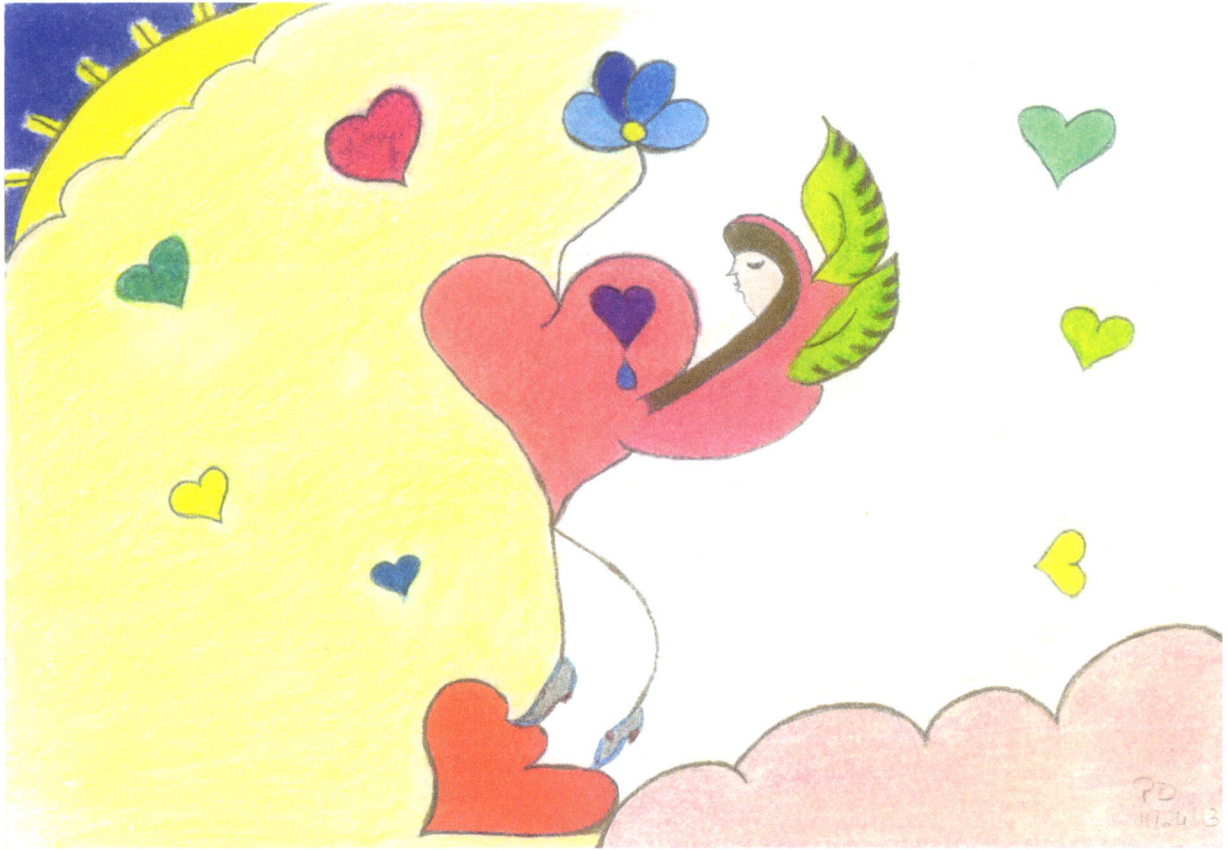

Heartful Flower Phoenix

Fly rising phoenix
Take my heart above the clouds
Heal it near the sun

When you feel unwanted or like an outcast, lift up your heart like a rising phoenix, and ride your heart fearlessly above the mesospheric clouds, where you wear your heart with wings in the sunlight and in the shade

Acknowledgments

God for being a constant presence which guides me in my work.

My husband, Ken Dellefield, who cherishes me and helps me to heal and to grow my heart.

My Father-in-law, Cal Dellefield, who saw the best in me as a writer and an artist.

Maryellen Dellefield for discovering the whimsical in my art.

Shambhala Meditation Center-San Diego, for the Dharma.

My best friend, Helen Wallace, who inspired me to write my first book.

My brother, Alex Turquieh, who was always encouraging me in my moments of doubt.

Mike Sager and The Sager Group for giving me a chance, for TSG Art Director Siori Kitajima for choosing the cover art and font for Being with Heart, and for copy editing by Leorah Gavidor.

Greg Shibley for additional copy editing and advice.

Jana Mazurkiewicz Meisarosh, at Yiddishland La Jolla, for giving Being with Heart initial exposure at her gallery.

About the Author

Pascale Dellefield is an author, artist, and the owner of Health and Peace Greetings, a greeting card company. Born in Beirut, Lebanon amid the chaos of war and civil unrest, she later moved to France and the U.S. and speaks four languages. A retired licensed Marriage and Family Therapist with a deep appreciation for diversity and social consciousness. She lives with her husband and two cats in San Diego.

About the Publisher

The Sager Group was founded in 1984. In 2012 it was chartered as a multimedia content brand, with the intent of empowering those who create art—an umbrella beneath which makers can pursue, and profit from, their craft directly, without gatekeepers. TSG publishes books; ministers to artists and provides modest grants; and produces documentary, feature, and commercial films. By harnessing the means of production, The Sager Group helps artists help themselves. For more information, please see TheSagerGroup.net.

More Books from The Sager Group

The Swamp: Deceit and Corruption in the CIA
An Elizabeth Petrov Thriller (Book 1)
by Jeff Grant

Chains of Nobility: Brotherhood of the Mamluks (Book 1-3)
by Brad Graft

Meeting Mozart: A Novel Drawn from the Secret Diaries of Lorenzo Da Ponte
by Howard Jay Smith

Death Came Swiftly: A Novel About the Tay Bridge Disaster of 1879
by Bill Abrams

A Boy and His Dog in Hell: And Other Stories
by Mike Sager

The Deadliest Man Alive: Count Dante, The Mob
and the War for American Martial Arts
by Benji Feldheim

Lifeboat No. 8: Surviving the Titanic
by Elizabeth Kaye

The Pope of Pot: And Other True Stories of Marijuana and Related High Jinks
by Mike Sager

See our entire library at TheSagerGroup.net

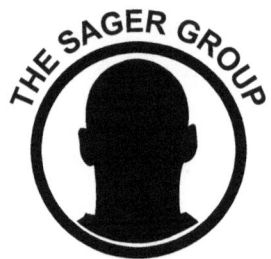

THE SAGER GROUP

Artifex Te Adiuva

www.ingramcontent.com/pod-product-compliance
Lightning Source LLC
Chambersburg PA
CBHW041105050426
42335CB00047B/161